Swine Flu

Swine Flu

How To Protect Your Health and Your Assets Against Pandemic

Mark Gordon MD

2009

Table of Contents

Introduction ix

Flu Pandemic Background 1

The facts about New H1N1 (Swine) Flu 5
    What are the signs and symptoms of this virus in
    people? 5
    How severe is illness associated with this new H1N1
    virus? 5
    How does this new H1N1 virus spread? 6
    How long can an infected person spread this virus to
    others? 6

Exposures Not Thought to Spread Swine Flu 7
    Is there a risk from drinking water? 7
    Can the new H1N1 flu virus be spread through water
    in swimming pools, spas, water parks, interactive
    fountains, and other treated recreational water
    venues? 7
    Can H1N1 influenza virus be spread at recreational
    water venues outside of the water? 8

Prevention & Treatment 9
    What can I do to protect myself from getting sick? . . . 9
    Take these everyday steps to protect your health: . . . 9
    Other important actions that you can take are: 9
    What is the best way to keep from spreading the virus
    through coughing or sneezing? 10
    What is the best technique for washing my hands to
    avoid getting the flu? 10
    What should I do if I get sick? .10

In children emergency warning signs that need urgent
medical attention include:.........................11
In adults, emergency warning signs that need urgent
medical attention include: 11
Are there medicines to treat infection with this new
virus?..11
Will face masks protect you from the flu? 12

Swine Flu's Vaccine.................................15

Contamination & Cleaning..........................17
How long can influenza virus remain viable on objects
(such as books and doorknobs)? 17
What kills influenza virus? 17
What surfaces are most likely to be sources of
contamination?...................................17
How should waste disposal be handled to prevent the
spread of influenza virus?........................17
What household cleaning should be done to prevent
the spread of influenza virus?....................18
How should linens, eating utensils and dishes of persons
infected with influenza virus be handled? 18

Response & Investigation..........................19
What are government agencies doing in response to
the outbreak? 19
What epidemiological investigations are taking place
in response to the recent outbreak?................19
Who is in charge of medicine in the Strategic National
Stockpile (SNS) once it is deployed?.............. 20

Will Your Travel Insurance Policy Cover Swine Flu Claims?.21

Watch out for swine flu scams....................... 25

Protect your business needs and financials........... 27
Allocate resources to protect your family during a
pandemic..................................... 27

Plan for the impact of a pandemic on your business. 28

Investments In Pandemic Influenza Preparedness Pay Off, But Are Threatened By Cuts In Federal Funding 29

How will the uninsured fare in swine flu outbreak? 31

Swine Flu Reports. 35

Introduction

Governments around the world are launching nationwide campaigns to inform the public about protective cautions against swine flu amid alarming reports from health agencies about the dangers posed by the virus.

So far, the majority of patients with the illness only reported fairly mild symptoms and enjoyed a good recovery.

Doctors believe, however, that a second, larger wave of infection during the traditional flu season of autumn and winter is possible. The World Health Organisation said that they will be on high alert, remaining on their guard. They reminded that the Spanish flu of 1918 surged in spring, disappeared in the summer months, and returned in the autumn of 1918 with a vengeance. The World Health Organization has long predicted a flu pandemic that will take more lives than the Spanish flu of 1918 wherein 20 to 40 million people perished.

Most dictionaries define pandemic as "an epidemic that is geographically widespread; occurring throughout a region or even throughout the world." Knowing this, what can you do to protect yourself and your family while the winds of pandemic are blowing in Mexico, US, Canada, Europe and Asia?

You either can wait for your government to devise a solution to protect you, or you can be proactive, and take the steps outlined below.

Flu Pandemic Background

I would like to go back to 1918 when the Spanish flu—caused by the same virus as swine flu—killed at least 50 million, many times more than the First World War. The Times journal has recently searched its archives to find out how Britain coped.

In February 1919, a reader has contacted the Editor of The Times to give advice on the most pressing matter of the day. "Sir, the simplest, easiest and cheapest precaution is to use salt water for gargling the throat and rinsing the nostrils," he says, before adding, for the benefit of those unfamiliar with nose-rinsing techniques, "fill the hollow of the hand and 'snuffle' the mixture."

For less sturdy readers, the Times doctor sums up the scientific consensus on defeating influenza: "The good effects of wine continue to be emphasised, and most agree in selecting port as the best of these," he says. An advertisement in the paper extols the benefits of mustard baths.

The Spanish flu pandemic that began in 1918 was the gravest medical disaster of the 20th century, comparable in scale only to the great plagues of the Middle Ages. Over the course of two winters, a third of the world's population became infected with the H1N1 flu virus—the same subtype as the current swine flu. Propagated by troops leaving the trenches and exacerbated by those cold winters, it spread to every continent. Woodrow Wilson, the US President, suffered from its effects while negotiating the Treaty of Versailles. Gustav Klimt, the Austrian painter, died in the first wave, aged 55. As with swine flu today, the virus seemed, unusually, to affect the young, fit and healthy.

By the summer of 1920 an estimated 50 million people had died. The toll from the preceding four years of bloody mechanised warfare in Russia and France, when the world's great powers had applied their finest minds to the challenge of killing each other's troops in the most efficient way possible, had been 15 million. For two years the failed attempts to control the disease and deal with its disastrous effects filled the pages of The Times.

The first report on "the Spanish epidemic", on June 3, 1918, was placed between progress updates on the Western Front and a speech in which President Wilson argued that "the spectacle of 20 nations battling against the forces of evil is evidence that Christ still rules in the hearts of men".

The article states: "The unknown disease which appeared in Madrid a fortnight ago spread with remarkable rapidity. Owing to its benign character it was at first, together with its victims, the subject of much badinage and pleasant writing in the newspapers. Today the complaint has passed the joking stage." The correspondent says that there have been 700 deaths in ten days.

Very soon, the epidemic would cease to be a foreign news story and 700 deaths in ten days would cease to be newsworthy. But before the pages of The Times became grim death-rolls—tables compiled across the country, recording city-by-city mortality—there was a "phoney war", a time for theorising and analysis.

"The man in the street, having been taught to take a keener interest in foreign affairs, discussed the news of the epidemic which spread with such surprising rapidity through Spain a few weeks ago, and cheerfully anticipated its arrival here," writes a Times columnist, who goes on to discuss possible causes of this mysterious illness. "He [the aforementioned "man in the street"] is sometimes inclined to believe it is really a form of pro-German influence—the "unseen hand" is popularly supposed to be carrying test tubes containing cultures of all the bacilli known to science, and many as yet unknown."

Any fantasies that the Spanish flu was really a German bio-weapon of last resort were soon lost, however, in the daily grind of dealing with yet more death even as the allies continued fighting on the Western Front. On November 7, 1918, four days before the end of the war, The Times published an article headlined "Rise in influenza death-roll". It follows the same template as dozens of articles in preceding months, and dozens in the months after. All that changes is the numbers.

Beneath the sub-heading "Over 7,000 last week" is a table with two columns simply labelled "last week" and "previous week". Prefixing these with the word "deaths" is no longer thought necessary. "London County, 2,458; London outer ring, 1,705; Sheffield, 465; Leicester, 260; Hull, 220 . . ."

Many of the deaths were preventable, had pre-NHS hospitals been able to cope. The Times observed in February 1919 that pneumonia cases were being turned away for lack of space: "We cannot afford to lose 100,000 of our young adult lives in 12 weeks because of the absence of hospital accommodation," the correspondent argued. Some wards had to close because all the nurses had flu.

Although popular remedies to combat flu may have involved mustard and Bovril, the world was still in a far better position to understand and mitigate the effects of the disease than it had been the last time it faced a pandemic. Advances in scientific understanding in the late 19th century meant that doctors understood the theory of germs and viruses and how they spread disease. Scientists still lacked the expertise to isolate and identify the pathogen but they knew how to avoid it. The Times advised its readers: "Infection is by contact, coughing, sneezing and even loud talking. The poison can be projected as far as 10ft from the infected host in this manner, hence the importance of over-crowding." As with swine flu in Mexico, the authorities recommended the use of masks and took measures to prevent large gatherings of people.

But a sterner early 20th-century medical establishment would have looked dimly on the measures taken last week in Devon, where a school was closed after a possible infection. "It has been necessary at some schools to close several departments, but that is for administrative reasons owing to a shortage of staff," Britain's chief medical officer told The Times in late 1918. "We are still of the opinion that the children are no more likely to fall victims of the illness in well-ventilated schools than they are running about the streets or packed together in picture theatres."

The Times's medical correspondent, meanwhile, grumbled that "the recent Tube strike has no doubt played a part in lowering public resistance . . . for long walks have had to be undertaken by tired-out men and women who . . . have been forced to face the ordeal on empty stomachs."

As the virus finally receded, taking with it much of the Great War generation, people searched for whatever lessons they could find. The Times reported on a lecture at the Royal Institute of Public Health, where Captain Thomas Carnwath argued for the general use of face masks. **"If people had learnt to use umbrellas, he did not see why they could not also learn to use masks," The Times wrote.**

The facts about New H1N1 (Swine) Flu

What are the signs and symptoms of this virus in people?

The symptoms of this new H1N1 flu virus in people are similar to the symptoms of seasonal flu and include fever, cough, sore throat, runny or stuffy nose, body aches, headache, chills and fatigue. A significant number of people who have been infected with this virus also have reported diarrhea and vomiting. Also, like seasonal flu, severe illnesses and death has occurred as a result of illness associated with this virus.

How severe is illness associated with this new H1N1 virus?

It's not known at this time how severe this virus will be in the general population. Researchers are studying the medical histories of people who have been infected with this virus to determine whether some people may be at greater risk from infection, serious illness or hospitalization from the virus. In seasonal flu, there are certain people that are at higher risk of serious flu-related complications. This includes people 65 years and older, children younger than five years old, pregnant women, and people of any age with chronic medical conditions. It's unknown at this time whether certain groups of people are at greater risk of serious flu-related complications from infection with this new virus. Researchers also are conducting laboratory studies to see if certain people might have natural immunity to this virus, depending on their age.

How does this new H1N1 virus spread?

Spread of this H1N1 virus is thought to be happening in the same way that seasonal flu spreads. Flu viruses are spread mainly from person to person through coughing or sneezing by people with influenza. Sometimes people may become infected by touching something with flu viruses on it and then touching their mouth or nose.

How long can an infected person spread this virus to others?

At the current time, Researchers believe that this virus has the same properties in terms of spread as seasonal flu viruses. With seasonal flu, studies have shown that people may be contagious from one day before they develop symptoms to up to 7 days after they get sick. Children, especially younger children, might potentially be contagious for longer periods. Researchers are studying the virus and its capabilities to try to learn more and will provide more information as it becomes available.

Exposures Not Thought to Spread Swine Flu

Is there a risk from drinking water?

Tap water that has been treated by conventional disinfection processes does not likely pose a risk for transmission of influenza viruses. Current drinking water treatment regulations provide a high degree of protection from viruses. No research has been completed on the susceptibility of the novel H1N1 flu virus to conventional drinking water treatment processes. However, recent studies have demonstrated that free chlorine levels typically used in drinking water treatment are adequate to inactivate highly pathogenic H5N1 avian influenza. It is likely that other influenza viruses such as novel H1N1 would also be similarly inactivated by chlorination. To date, there have been no documented human cases of influenza caused by exposure to influenza-contaminated drinking water.

Can the new H1N1 flu virus be spread through water in swimming pools, spas, water parks, interactive fountains, and other treated recreational water venues?

Influenza viruses infect the human upper respiratory tract. There has never been a documented case of influenza virus infection associated with water exposure. Recreational water that has been treated at CDC recommended disinfectant levels does not likely pose a risk for transmission of influenza viruses. No research has been completed on

Mark Gordon MD

the susceptibility of the H1N1 influenza virus to chlorine and other disinfectants used in swimming pools, spas, water parks, interactive fountains, and other treated recreational venues. However, recent studies have demonstrated that free chlorine levels recommended by CDC (1–3 parts per million [ppm or mg/L] for pools and 2–5 ppm for spas) are adequate to disinfect avian influenza A (H5N1) virus. It is likely that other influenza viruses such as novel H1N1 virus would also be similarly disinfected by chlorine.

Can H1N1 influenza virus be spread at recreational water venues outside of the water?

Yes, recreational water venues are no different than any other group setting. The spread of this novel H1N1 flu is thought to be happening in the same way that seasonal flu spreads. Flu viruses are spread mainly from person to person through coughing or sneezing of people with influenza. Sometimes people may become infected by touching something with flu viruses on it and then touching their mouth or nose.

Prevention & Treatment

What can I do to protect myself from getting sick?

There is no vaccine available right now to protect against this new H1N1 virus. There are everyday actions that can help prevent the spread of germs that cause respiratory illnesses like influenza.

Take these everyday steps to protect your health:

- Cover your nose and mouth with a tissue when you cough or sneeze. Throw the tissue in the trash after you use it.
- Wash your hands often with soap and water, especially after you cough or sneeze. Alcohol-based hand cleaners are also effective.
- Avoid touching your eyes, nose or mouth. Germs spread this way.
- Try to avoid close contact with sick people.
- Stay home if you are sick for 7 days after your symptoms begin or until you have been symptom-free for 24 hours, whichever is longer. This is to keep from infecting others and spreading the virus further.

Other important actions that you can take are:

- Follow public health advice regarding school closures, avoiding crowds and other social distancing measures.
- Be prepared in case you get sick and need to stay home for a week or so; a supply of over-the-counter medicines, alcohol-based hand rubs, tissues

and other related items might could be useful and help avoid the need to make trips out in public while you are sick and contagious.

What is the best way to keep from spreading the virus through coughing or sneezing?

If you are sick, limit your contact with other people as much as possible. If you are sick, stay home for 7 days after your symptoms begin or until you have been symptom-free for 24 hours, whichever is longer. Cover your mouth and nose with a tissue when coughing or sneezing. Put your used tissue in the waste basket. Then, clean your hands, and do so every time you cough or sneeze.

What is the best technique for washing my hands to avoid getting the flu?

Washing your hands often will help protect you from germs. Wash with soap and water or clean with alcohol-based hand cleaner. It is recommended that when you wash your hands—with soap and warm water—that you wash for 15 to 20 seconds. When soap and water are not available, alcohol-based disposable hand wipes or gel sanitizers may be used. You can find them in most supermarkets and drugstores. If using gel, rub your hands until the gel is dry. The gel doesn't need water to work; the alcohol in it kills the germs on your hands.

What should I do if I get sick?

If you live in areas where people have been identified with new H1N1 flu and become ill with influenza-like symptoms, including fever, body aches, runny or stuffy nose, sore throat, nausea, or vomiting or diarrhea, you should stay home and avoid contact with other people, except to seek medical care.

If you have severe illness or you are at high risk for flu complications, contact your health care provider or seek medical care. Your health care provider will determine whether flu testing or treatment is needed

If you become ill and experience any of the following warning signs, seek emergency medical care.

In children emergency warning signs that need urgent medical attention include:

- Fast breathing or trouble breathing
- Bluish or gray skin color
- Not drinking enough fluids
- Severe or persistent vomiting
- Not waking up or not interacting
- Being so irritable that the child does not want to be held
- Flu-like symptoms improve but then return with fever and worse cough

In adults, emergency warning signs that need urgent medical attention include:

- Difficulty breathing or shortness of breath
- Pain or pressure in the chest or abdomen
- Sudden dizziness
- Confusion
- Severe or persistent vomiting
- Flu-like symptoms improve but then return with fever and worse cough

Are there medicines to treat infection with this new virus?

YesDoctors recommend the use of oseltamivir or zanamivir for the treatment and/or prevention of infection with the new H1N1 flu virus. Antiviral drugs are prescription medicines (pills, liquid or an inhaler) that fight against the flu by keeping flu viruses from reproducing in your body. If you get sick, antiviral drugs can make your illness milder and make you feel better faster. They may also prevent serious flu complications. During the current outbreak, the priority use for influenza antiviral drugs during is to treat severe influenza illness.

Will face masks protect you from the flu?

According to CBCnews, in the aftermath of the SARS outbreak in 2003, the Public Health Agency of Canada asked a panel of medical experts for guidance on how flu is transmitted and how best to protect against infection.

Their report concluded that the scientific evidence remains unclear about how precisely flu is spread and what role exposure to bigger or smaller virus particles plays in transmission. It found that flu viruses are mainly transmitted over short distances and that more people become infected by inhaling viruses than by touching contaminated surfaces.

The report was produced by the Council of Canadian Academies, chaired by Dr. Donald Low, microbiologist in chief at Mount Sinai Hospital in Toronto.

One of the questions the panel considered was whether face masks would offer protection in the event of a pandemic.

The verdict: yes, to an extent.

The report says a face mask—or personal protective respiratory equipment—is the final layer of protection when exposure to an infected person is required, or unavoidable. The primary elements of protection are "engineering and administrative controls."

Engineering controls include physical controls such as ventilation requirements in buildings, and relative humidity and temperature controls. Administrative controls are measures that individuals handle, such as handwashing, covering your mouth when you sneeze or cough or seeking medical care when you're sick.

A protective mask, the report says, can offer protection, but there's no evidence inexpensive surgical masks can protect against flu virus particles small enough to be inhaled into the lower respiratory tract or the lungs. The report also finds that it's unclear how effective surgical masks are in blocking flu virus particles that are bigger and therefore likely to settle in the nose and throat of an exposed person.

Not all masks are created equally, either. Surgical masks—the kind your dental hygienist might use while inflicting a cleaning on you—offer some help, but they won't filter out smaller particles and don't provide a good seal.

If you're in the market for a mask, don't go to the hardware store and pick up one that you'd use while sanding drywall. Covering your mouth and nose with a bandana won't do you much good either.

The best bet for protective masks are what are referred to as "N95 respirators," a commonly used term in Canada that refers to NIOSH-certified, disposable, particulate-filtering, half-facepiece respirators.

Not all high-quality masks are labeled N95. Health Canada said masks should offer protection equivalent to N95 to be considered effective. Such masks should:

- Filter particles one micron in size or smaller.
- Have a 95 per cent filter efficiency.
- Provide a tight facial seal (less than 10% leak).

Authorities tested three types of N95 masks in the wake of the SARS outbreak in 2003. Each filtered out between 97 per cent and 99.7 per cent of all the virus-like particles.

The report further concluded that:

- N95 respirators protect against the inhalation of nasopharyngeal, tracheobronchial and alveolar sized particles.
- Surgical masks worn by an infected person may play a role in the prevention of influenza transmission by reducing the amount of infectious material that is expelled into the environment.
- Both surgical masks and N95 respirators offer a physical barrier to contact with contaminated

      hands and ballistic trajectory particles, such as particles expelled by a sneeze or a cough.

- The efficiency of the filters of surgical masks to block penetration of alveolar and tracheobronchial sized particles is highly variable. When combined with the inability to ensure a sealed fit, these factors suggest that surgical masks offer no significant protection against the inhalation of alveolar and tracheobronchial sized particles.

Health officials say masks can help, but unless the person wearing the mask can ensure a sealed fit, the mask will offer no significant protection. This can be more of a problem for children or men with beards.

Swine Flu's Vaccine

The efforts are under way to create a seed vaccine strain which could then be grown in bulk by manufacturers. Scientists need a steady hand to drill a hole in a hen's egg. This is the first step in the creation of a vaccine against the swine flu virus. If exposed to the virus, the immune system will destroy the invader before it can cause illness.

No-one should expect a swine flu vaccine to be available before the Autumn. In fact most of us will have to wait a lot longer. Around 300 million doses of seasonal flu vaccine are produced globally each year.

The vaccine includes three different strains of human flu so each dose takes three eggs to produce. If manufacturers switched to producing a single pandemic strain vaccine, they might feasibly triple the number of doses to around 900 million. But it may not be that simple.

We do not know how well the virus will grow in eggs or how much antigen will be needed to create an effective vaccine. It may require two injections to provide adequate immunity.

Contamination & Cleaning

How long can influenza virus remain viable on objects (such as books and doorknobs)?

Studies have shown that influenza virus can survive on environmental surfaces and can infect a person for up to 2-8 hours after being deposited on the surface.

What kills influenza virus?

Influenza virus is destroyed by heat (167-212°F [75-100°C]). In addition, several chemical germicides, including chlorine, hydrogen peroxide, detergents (soap), iodophors (iodine-based antiseptics), and alcohols are effective against human influenza viruses if used in proper concentration for a sufficient length of time. For example, wipes or gels with alcohol in them can be used to clean hands. The gels should be rubbed into hands until they are dry.

What surfaces are most likely to be sources of contamination?

Germs can be spread when a person touches something that is contaminated with germs and then touches his or her eyes, nose, or mouth. Droplets from a cough or sneeze of an infected person move through the air. Germs can be spread when a person touches respiratory droplets from another person on a surface like a desk, for example, and then touches their own eyes, mouth or nose before washing their hands.

How should waste disposal be handled to prevent the spread of influenza virus?

To prevent the spread of influenza virus, it is recommended that tissues and other disposable items used by an infected person be thrown in the trash. Additionally, persons should wash their hands with soap and water after touching used tissues and similar waste.

What household cleaning should be done to prevent the spread of influenza virus?

To prevent the spread of influenza virus it is important to keep surfaces (especially bedside tables, surfaces in the bathroom, kitchen counters and toys for children) clean by wiping them down with a household disinfectant according to directions on the product label.

How should linens, eating utensils and dishes of persons infected with influenza virus be handled?

Linens, eating utensils, and dishes belonging to those who are sick do not need to be cleaned separately, but importantly these items should not be shared without washing thoroughly first.

Linens (such as bed sheets and towels) should be washed by using household laundry soap and tumbled dry on a hot setting. Individuals should avoid "hugging" laundry prior to washing it to prevent contaminating themselves. Individuals should wash their hands with soap and water or alcohol-based hand rub immediately after handling dirty laundry.

Eating utensils should be washed either in a dishwasher or by hand with water and soap.

Response & Investigation

What are government agencies doing in response to the outbreak?

Government has implemented its emergency response. The goals are to reduce transmission and illness severity, and provide information to help health care providers, public health officials and the public address the challenges posed by the new virus. Government continues to issue new interim guidance for clinicians and public health professionals. In addition, Government's Division of the Strategic National Stockpile (SNS) continues to send antiviral drugs, personal protective equipment, and respiratory protection devices to all 50 states and U.S. territories to help them respond to the outbreak.

What epidemiological investigations are taking place in response to the recent outbreak?

Government works very closely with state and local officials in areas where human cases of new H1N1 flu infections have been identified. In California and Texas, where EpiAid teams have been deployed, many epidemiological activities are taking place or planned including:

- Active surveillance in the counties where infections in humans have been identified;
- Studies of health care workers who were exposed to patients infected with the virus to see if they became infected;

- Studies of households and other contacts of people who were confirmed to have been infected to see if they became infected;
- Study of a public high school where three confirmed human cases of H1N1 flu occurred to see if anyone became infected and how much contact they had with a confirmed case; and
- Study to see how long a person with the virus infection sheds the virus.

Who is in charge of medicine in the Strategic National Stockpile (SNS) once it is deployed?

Local health officials have full control of SNS medicine once supplies are deployed to a city, state, or territory. Federal, state, and local community planners are working together to ensure that SNS medicines will be delivered to the affected area as soon as possible. Many cities, states, and territories have already received SNS supplies. After Government sends medicine to a state or city, control and distribution of the supply is at the discretion of that state or local health department. Most states and cities also have their own medicines that they can access to treat infected persons.

Will Your Travel Insurance Policy Cover Swine Flu Claims?

As with all insurance-related questions, the answer lies in the fine print of your policy. Some travel insurance policies include clauses that exclude claims related to known events, epidemics or pandemics. As of April 24, 2009, swine flu is a "known event," according to the travel insurance providers we surveyed. Therefore, policies purchased after this date may not cover claims related to swine flu.

All fine print has exceptions, though. In most cases, "cancel for any reason" coverage will protect you even if you bought your policy after April 24. Still, it's best to read your policy carefully, especially if you have already bought coverage.

Normally, buying travel insurance is a great way to protect your vacation investment. During this swine flu outbreak, special conditions apply.

Travel insurance providers are approaching the swine flu crisis in a variety of ways. For example:

Travel Guard's "Cancel for Any Reason" coverage is offered as an upgrade to some Travel Guard trip insurance plans. If you purchase this upgrade, Travel Guard will reimburse you up to 75 percent of your trip cancellation penalty as long as you cancel your trip at least 48 hours before departure. Reimbursement percentage depends on the coverage offered under the travel insurance plan you purchase.

Travel Guard also offers telephone assistance to travelers seeking information and referrals for swine flu. If you believe you are exhibiting symptoms of swine flu, you can call 866-644-6811 in the U.S. and Canada or 715-295-1209 collect from overseas. Travel Guard also offers swine flu information on its U.S. and Canadian websites.

Access America / Mondial Assistance says on their (combined) website that policies purchased on or after April 24, 2009, will not cover any swine flu-related claims. Some policies sold before April 24, 2009, may not cover swine flu claims due to specific policy exclusions for epidemics or pandemics.

Most Travel Protection policies cover trip cancellation if you are being treated by a doctor for a particular illness that was contracted after you purchased your travel insurance policy. It is recommended that travelers who want the flexibility of canceling a trip regardless of reason should look for a company that offers 'Cancel for Any Reason' policies. Fear of traveling, or government advisories against travel, are not covered reasons under the majority of travel insurance policies, but would be covered under a 'Cancel for Any Reason' policy. Consumers should be aware that most 'Cancel for Any Reason' policies pay a sliding scale of benefits in the event of cancellation."

As conditions change, your best bet is to contact your travel insurance provider for up-to-date information.

If you are planning to travel but have not yet purchased travel insurance, you should carefully consider your feelings about traveling during a pandemic. Most travel insurance policies will not cover you if you cancel your trip because you are worried about a particular disease unless you have purchased "Cancel for Any Reason" coverage. Even if your airline will not fly into a swine flu area, your travel insurance policy may not cover your situation. Contact your travel insurance provider before buying a policy if, after reading the entire policy, you still have questions.

In situations where you are requesting that a claim be paid, it is always best to conduct your business in writing, either by email or by traceable traditional mailing methods. If you do not receive a prompt reply to your correspondence, consider resending the letter or claim form, this time sending a copy to a senior executive of the travel insurance company. Keep a log of all correspondence, including emails and telephone calls, just in case.

Watch out for swine flu scams

It didn't take scammers long to latch on to the latest hot-button topic to try to make a quick buck. Scams built on fears of swine flu are proliferating quickly across the Internet.

The U.S. Computer Emergency Readiness Team issued an alert this week warning of a number of e-mail scams related to the swine flu. The attacks arrive via an unsolicited e-mail message typically containing a subject line related to the swine flu.

"These e-mail messages may contain a link or an attachment. If users click on this link or open the attachment, they may be directed to a phishing Web site or exposed to malicious code," the alert said.

US-CERT encourages users to take the following measures to protect themselves:

- Filter spam.
- Don't trust unsolicited e-mail.
- Treat e-mail attachments with caution.
- Don't click links in e-mail messages.
- Install antivirus software and keep it up-to-date.
- Install a personal firewall and keep it up-to-date.
- Configure your e-mail client for security.

To stay informed about swine flu, US-CERT says you should rely on trusted sources of information, such as the U.S. Centers for Disease Control.

Also, be highly skeptical of unknown Web sites with the words "swine flu" in the domain name. Online security firm F-Secure reports that dozens of new swine flu domain names

Mark Gordon MD

were registered in the last few days. F-Secure said some of these sites are already offering ways to "protect your family from this crazy flu."

Protect your business needs and financials

Even if swine flu is not making you sneeze, it could still be making you sick in other ways. The drop in stocks is the last thing investors need as stockholders wait out this period of economic recovery. Airlines were the first to feel the pinch, as they prepared for less travel in general and fewer trips to Mexico especially.

Allocate resources to protect your family during a pandemic

Take out some money: Keep extra cash at home. If there is a pandemic, getting money from ATMs may become difficult. Banks ran scenarios of what could happen if there were a pandemic flu outbreak in response to the H5N1 bird flu virus a few years back. One of the findings was that ATMs could quickly run dry of cash as many workers who were supposed to replenish them called in sick or couldn't come to work to take care of family members who were sick. This could also easily extend to other necessities.

Ensure you have access to the credit should you need it: A stay in a hospital could spell financial ruin. With many people out of a job and no longer covered by health insurance, the cost for treatment could be massive. Even a mild case of swine flu could end up costing hundreds of dollars in doctors' visits, treatments and tests, and lost work hours.

Ensure availability of sufficient and accessible infection control supplies (e.g.hand-hygiene products, tissues and receptacles for their disposal) in all business locations.

Ensure availability of medical consultation and advice for emergency response.

Plan for the impact of a pandemic on your business

Identify a pandemic coordinator and/or team with defined roles and responsibilities for preparedness and response planning. The planning process should include input from labor representatives.

Identify essential employees and other critical inputs (e.g. raw materials, suppliers, sub-contractor services/ products, and logistics) required to maintain business operations by location and function during a pandemic.

Train and prepare ancillary workforce (e.g. contractors, employees in other job titles/descriptions, retirees).

Develop and plan for scenarios likely to result in an increase or decrease in demand for your products and/or services during a pandemic (e.g. effect of restriction on mass gatherings, need for hygiene supplies).

Determine potential impact of a pandemic on company business financials using multiple possible scenarios that affect different product lines and/or production sites.

Determine potential impact of a pandemic on business-related domestic and international travel (e.g. quarantines, border closures).

Find up-to-date, reliable pandemic information from community public health, emergency management, and other sources and make sustainable links.

Establish an emergency communications plan and revise periodically. This plan includes identification of key contacts (with back-ups), chain of communications (including suppliers and customers), and processes for tracking and communicating business and employee status.

Implement an exercise/drill to test your plan, and revise periodically.

Investments In Pandemic Influenza Preparedness Pay Off, But Are Threatened By Cuts In Federal Funding

"States have made important progress toward preparing for their unique roles in combating an influenza pandemic but have much more to do," according to a report submitted to the Homeland Security Council.

"The Association of State and Territorial Health Officials (ASTHO) supports that finding," said Executive Director Paul E. Jarris, MD, MBA. "States have made tremendous progress toward combating pandemic influenza since the threat was first identified and funding was made available in 2005. Continued progress is being jeopardized, however, by reductions in federal funding."

Federal funding for state and territorial pandemic preparedness ended in August 2008 and is not included in the FY09 budget. In addition, overall federal funding for preparedness activities has been cut by 25 percent since 2005.

"States are not in a position to replace the federal funding," said Dr. Judy Monroe, ASTHO President and Indiana State Health Commissioner. "Across the board, states and their health departments are experiencing devastating budget cuts. Reductions in federal preparedness funding for pandemics or other hazards will not only prevent additional advances, but will erode the ability of current programs to protect our citizens."

For example, important strides in preparing to care for vulnerable populations during a pandemic have been made. The significant time and money invested in those preparations will be lost and the people they protect will be put at further risk if funds to implement the plans are cut.

"Public health agencies thoroughly understand the complex and devastating effects of pandemics," said Jarris. "We're closely watching Egypt and China, where the latest avian flu outbreaks are occurring. The number of cases ending in death is alarming; in some areas reaching over 65%. We can't let that happen in the United States."

Protecting America's health and effectively responding to emergencies, whether pandemics or terrorist attacks, requires sustained commitment and financial support. As today's report notes, "Preparedness is dynamic rather than static." Whether it improves or deteriorates over time depends on investment and commitment.

How will the uninsured fare in swine flu outbreak?

It has been reported that Swine flu could shine a glaring light on the best and worst about American-style health care.

At top labs, scientists are optimistic they can make a vaccine that's effective against the new virus. But in a country where one in seven people lack medical insurance, doctors worry that some individuals won't get needed protection because of cost.

It could leave the rest of society more vulnerable.

In a flu epidemic, the uninsured face the worst options: flooding the emergency rooms or self-medicating with cold preparations and hoping for the best. Many might not be aware they can also go to a federally-funded community health center and see a doctor or nurse for little or no cost.

Helping the estimated 50 million uninsured will mean more than just paying for their health care. For example, if they're here as illegal immigrants, should taxpayers still cover the costs?

Public health experts say obstacles to getting medical attention are counterproductive if you're trying to stop an infectious disease in a highly mobile society like the United States.

"The person I'm most worried about is the one who decides to delay getting care, and does it in such a way that they infect others or put themselves at greater risk," said

Mark Gordon MD

Dr. Georges Benjamin, executive director of the American Public Health Association. "To have an epidemic with millions of people who may not go to the doctor because they can't afford to pay remains one of the unique challenges of our system."

Lawmakers are already proposing fixes. The big health care overhaul Congress is working on probably won't be ready if a bad flu strikes later this year.

Senators have introduced legislation to pay for temporary medical treatment for uninsured people during a public health emergency. It could be a natural disaster such as an earthquake or hurricane, a bioterror attack, or a medical emergency such as a flu pandemic.

"We can't afford to have barriers that keep people from getting care when an epidemic is sweeping the community," they say.

Some have proposed to offer all individuals a free flu shot each year.

The Obama administration has not taken a position on either bill. But it has started shipping anti-flu medicines to community health centers, which provide basic medical care to the uninsured.

Trust for America's Health, a public health group that has focused on pandemic flu preparedness, is supporting the Durbin-Capps bill.

"During a public health emergency, the federal government would step in and take care of the needs of the people who are affected by that emergency," said Jeff Levi, executive director of the group. "Health care providers would not be left holding the bag for people who are uninsured. It will be a 'win' for individuals because they'll be able to get the care they need."

Many details of the legislation are still being worked out. Government coverage would be limited to treatment for problems that are related to the public emergency.

Dealing with immigrants could be one of the most difficult issues.

The uninsured are mostly native born. But immigrants are more than twice as likely to be uninsured as people born here.

When Congress was under Republican control it sharply restricted safety net benefits for immigrants, even legal ones. The Democratic-controlled Congress reversed that trend for legal immigrants when it expanded health insurance earlier this year for children in low-income families.

It would be another issue to cover illegal immigrants, even if only for a short time. But since Mexico is the epicenter of the outbreak, some experts say that may be prudent.

"We don't want to have a policy that drives people underground," Benjamin said. "It's better to have them present for care so that they don't put anybody else at risk."

Swine Flu Reports

On May 1 2009, flu reached 11 countries. Governments closed schools, planned for vaccine production and tapped emergency stockpiles of antiviral medicine.

Genetic tests have confirmed more than 331 people have the strain originally labeled swine flu, according to the World Health Organization's Web site. Hundreds more cases are suspected in New York, Mexico, Australia and New Zealand. The WHO said thousands of samples from sick patients are backlogged for testing, and disease trackers are looking at whether an outbreak in Spain should trigger a declaration of a pandemic.

The Geneva-based health agency raised its six-tier alert to 5 on April 29 and said a move to the next and final level, for the world's first influenza pandemic since 1968, may soon be made. The WHO urged countries to make final preparations against a disease that may sweep across the globe, preying on a world population that has no natural immunity to the new virus.

"What the public health community can and must do is provide the very best information," Michael Osterholm, director of the Center for Infectious Disease Research and Policy, at the University of Minnesota, in Minneapolis, said in a telephone interview. "We make general guideline recommendations, but it's all local leaders who decide."

Fort Worth, Texas, closed 144 public schools with 80,000 students after one child came down with flu. Citigroup Inc. disinfected a New York office building when a worker became ill, and as many as 400,000 pigs are being slaughtered in Egypt.

Pork is Safe

The flu infections in people aren't related to exposure to pigs, and properly prepared pork is safe to eat, said Keiji Fukuda, WHO assistant director-general for health security and environment.

As the number of people sick with flu continued to rise, an outbreak in Spain may show the virus is establishing itself beyond Mexico and the U.S., approaching the WHO's definition of a pandemic. The agency needs evidence of sustained human-to- human transmission outside North America to declare the outbreak a pandemic.

Spain confirmed 13 cases, including one person who hadn't been to Mexico. The WHO raised the alert to level 5 after swine flu took root in New York. It was the second elevation this week.

A phase 5 warning is "a strong signal that a pandemic is imminent" with little time left for preparation, according to the Web site of the WHO, an agency of the United Nations. It's based on the determination that the disease is established in communities in two countries in the same WHO region.

Schools Closed

In the U.S., at least 298 schools closed, leaving parents to find other arrangements for 172,000 students, according to the Education Department. The Centers for Disease Control and Prevention, a U.S. agency based in Atlanta, raised its flu count to 109, including a 22-month-old child who died April 2/ at a Houston hospital.

A note sent to U.S. Department of Homeland Security employees and obtained by Bloomberg News said masks must be worn by all workers who come within six feet (1.8 meters) of people known to have or who are suspected of having the virus. The department's workers include customs and border officers and airport baggage screeners.

A Citigroup employee in New York and a World Bank employee in Maryland were preliminarily diagnosed with the flu. One of Barack Obama's aides who traveled to Mexico as part of last month's presidential trip, along with his family, showed symptoms.

Word Bank Aid

The World Bank yesterday gave $25.6 million to Mexico for antiviral drugs, medical supplies and equipment to test for swine flu. The payment is the first of $205 million the World Bank pledged on April 26 to help Mexico cope with the outbreak, according to the bank's news release.

Margaret Chan, WHO's director-general, said travel restrictions won't slow the flu. Countries should ready emergency plans, she said on April 29.

Batches of seed virus are being developed for potential vaccine production, according to WHO. Paris-based Sanofi-Aventis SA, Baxter International Inc. of Deerfield, Illinois, and GlaxoSmithKline Plc of London are talking with world health authorities about how to make a vaccine.

Production of shots against seasonal flu will be completed before pandemic flu vaccine production begins, if that decision is made, said Richard Besser, acting head of the CDC.

Drugs Deployed

The CDC deployed antiviral drugs from the U.S. stockpile to 9 of 11 states with confirmed cases, Besser said. Shipments to the two other states should be finished by May 3. The CDC is adding more communications staff and equipment to field 4,000 calls, 2,000 e-mails and up to 8 million visits to its Web site a day, he said.

The U.S. will spend $251 million to buy 13 million courses of antiviral treatments to replenish its stockpile, said Health and Human Services Secretary Kathleen Sebelius. The White House said 20 states have probable or confirmed cases.

Jose Cordova, the health minister in Mexico, where the toll is highest, said yesterday the number of H1N1 flu cases confirmed by laboratory tests climbed to 312 from 260, and the death toll remained at 12. Deaths from the virus will probably rise, he said.

Mark Gordon MD

A "worrisome sign from Mexico was the relatively young healthy adults" succumbing to the virus, Anne Schuchat, interim deputy director of the CDC science and public health program, said yesterday in Congress. She said the average age of those in the U.S. confirmed to have the flu is 22.

Spain Question

The WHO's statistics, which lag behind those reported by national and local agencies, showed confirmed cases in the U.S., Mexico, Canada, Austria, Germany, the Netherlands, Switzerland, Israel, Spain, the U.K. and New Zealand. Only the U.S. and Mexico have confirmed deaths, according to the WHO.

Disease trackers are trying to determine whether the new virus, known formally as influenza A (H1N1), is spreading efficiently in Spain, said Dick Thompson, a spokesman for WHO.

Among the 13 cases in Spain, at least one patient hadn't traveled to Mexico, Thompson said. One case "confirmed to us that there's some community transmission beginning," he said. "The virus is becoming established in another area. It's this new single case that is especially worrying."

The last pandemic, 41 years ago, killed 1 million people and was mild compared with the global outbreak of 1918, which may have killed as many as 50 million.

Texas, California

President Obama asked Congress this week for $1.5 billion to battle an outbreak, and said parents should plan for school closings. Texas Governor Rick Perry declared a disaster, a "pre-emptive" measure to facilitate emergency preparations and seek federal reimbursement. California Governor Arnold Schwarzenegger declared a state of emergency.

New Zealand today said the number of people suspected as having the flu is 116, and said it has four laboratory-confirmed cases and 12 probable cases. In total, there are 388 people in isolation and receiving medication, said

38

the health ministry in New Zealand, the only Asia-Pacific nation with WHO-confirmed cases.

South Korea said it found two more probable flu cases, taking its total to three. Japan said test results for a 17- year-old male who visited Canada may be available today to determine if he's the nation's first swine-flu case. China began checking the body temperatures of travelers from the U.S.

Seasonal Strains

The three main seasonal flu strains—H3N2, H1N1 and type- B—cause 250,000 to 500,000 deaths a year globally, according to WHO. The new flu's symptoms are similar, including fever and coughing, nausea and vomiting, according to the CDC. It appears to be causing more diarrhea than seasonal flu, WHO said.

The U.S. can expect more hospitalizations and deaths, Sebelius said. Authorities advised hand-washing, hygiene and staying home if sick as the most effective ways to control the outbreak.

A Marine is recovering after being confirmed as having the virus, and another 37 Marines are being "watched and tested" at a base with 15,000 personnel in 29 Palms, California, Marine Corps Commandant General James Conway said at the Pentagon.

References

Health Archives
Medical and Epidemiology Journals
US Government news
Healthcare news
Medical Insurance news
The Time

www.ingramcontent.com/pod-product-compliance
Lightning Source LLC
Chambersburg PA
CBHW060650290526
45793CB00001B/474